Keto Chaffle Recipes Cookbook

The Perfect Guide to do Effortless and Enchanting Recipes with your Waffle Maker

Reyhan Hoque

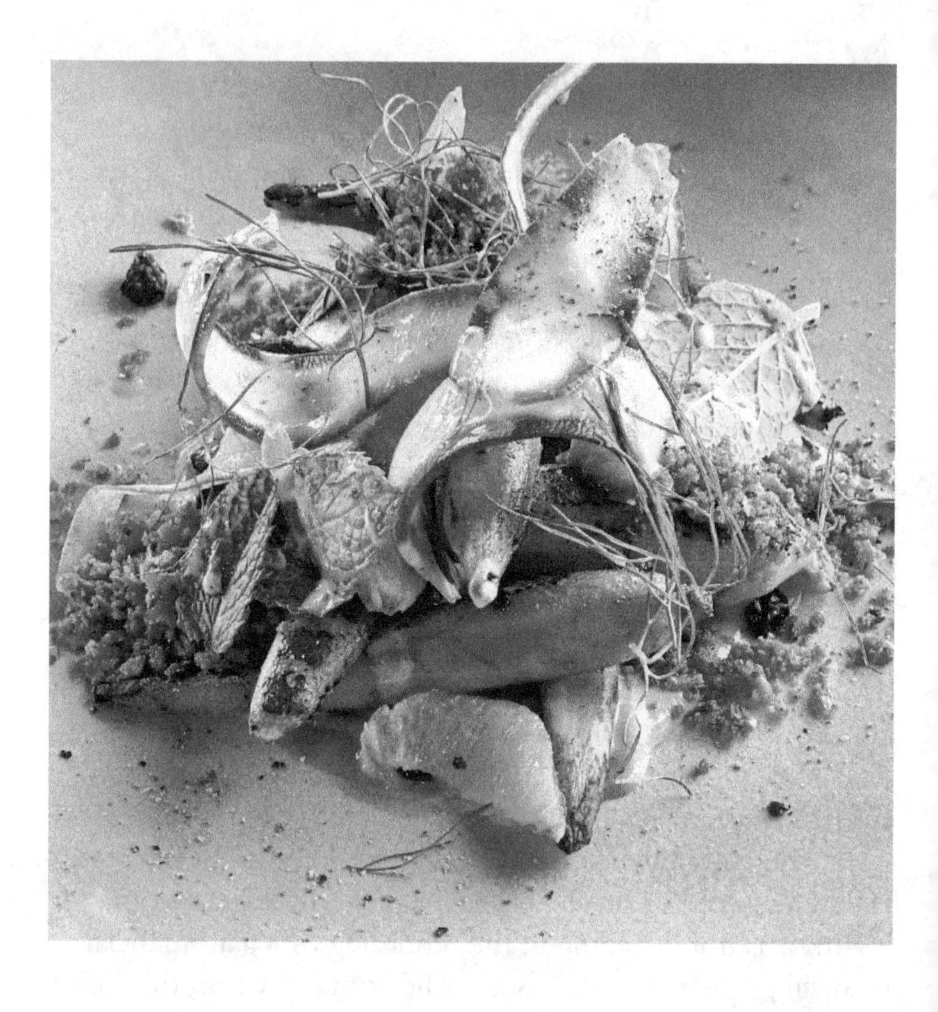

TABLE OF CONTENTS

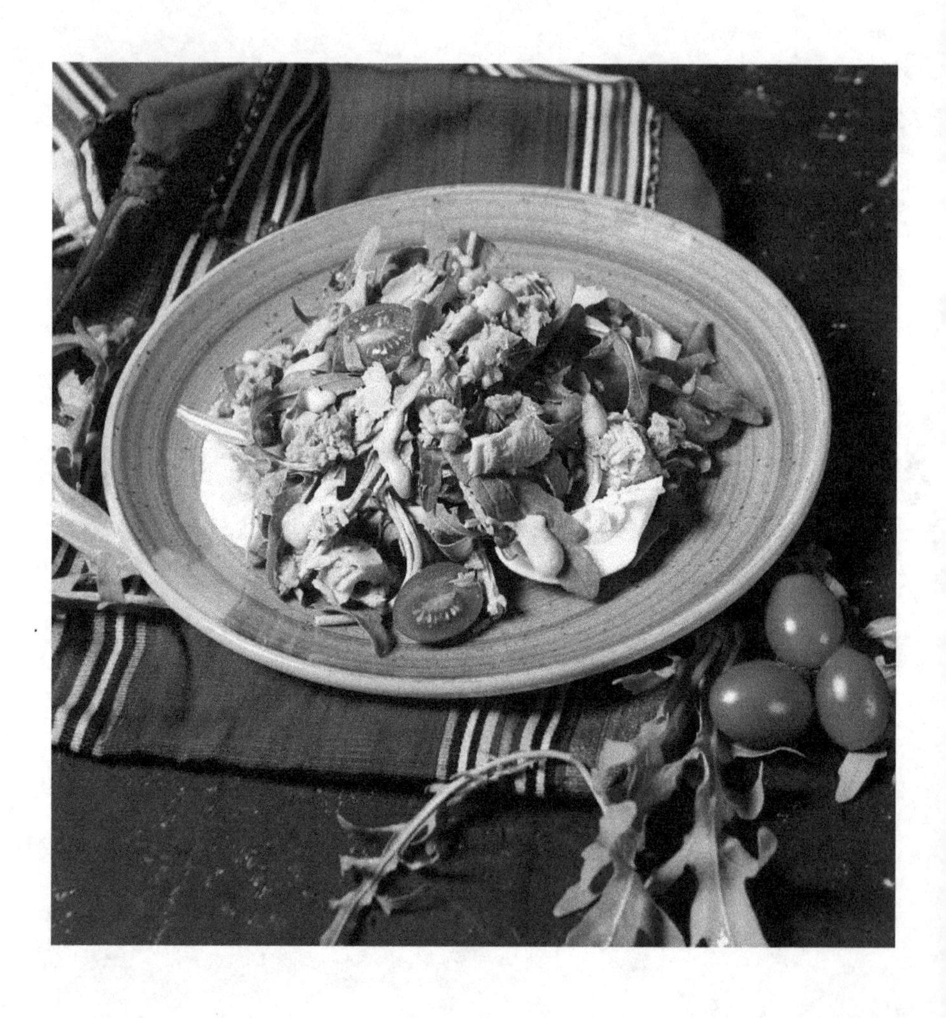

INTRODUCTION

A chaffle, or cheese waffle, is an egg and cheese keto waffle. Chaffles become a popular snack of keto / low-carb. Chaffle is made with coconut and pumpkin, making it a healthy low-carb alternative for anyone looking to lose weight. The chaffle helps stabilize blood sugar levels so the body has an easier time sensing when food is needed. The keto chaffle contains no calories or carbs, making it an ideal tool for anyone looking to lose or maintain their weight.

What is this keto Chaffle recipe in the world that has overtaken and conquered the keto community? Simply put, it's a cheese and egg waffle. There have been various variants in Facebook groups since the original recipe came out

How to make crispy chaffle

First off, beat one egg in a mixing bowl until you achieve the desired consistency and add ½ cup of finely shredded mozzarella cheese. Preheat the mini waffle iron then pour the mixture into it

If you find the taste too eggy, you can add a tablespoon of almond flour or any keto-friendly flour like coconut flour, psyllium husk flour, ground flax seed and the like. You can also top it with sugar free syrup and butter.

You can also try other kinds of cheese to see what will make your taste buds happier.

If you want it crunchier, you have to sprinkle shredded cheese on the waffle maker first and let it melt for half a minute before adding the mixture.

This is just the classic chaffle though. Remember that you can be creative with it and possibilities are endless!

Chaffles can be used for hamburger bun, hotdog bun, sandwich and pizza crust. You can also make it sweet or savory.

11 Tips to Make Chaffles

- **Preheat Well:** Yes! It sounds obvious to preheat the waffle iron before usage. However, preheating the iron moderately will not get your chaffles as crispy as you will like. The best way to preheat before cooking is to ensure that the iron is very hot.

- **Not-So-Cheesy:** Will you prefer to have your chaffles less cheesy? Then, use mozzarella cheese.
- **Not-So Eggy**: If you aren't comfortable with the smell of eggs in your chaffles, try using egg whites instead of egg yolks or whole eggs.
- **To Shred or to Slice:** Many recipes call for shredded cheese when making chaffles, but I find sliced cheeses to offer crispier pieces. While I stick with mostly shredded cheese for convenience's sake, be at ease to use sliced cheese in the same quantity. When using sliced cheeses, arrange two to four pieces in the waffle iron, top with the beaten eggs, and some slices of the cheese. Cover and cook until crispy.
- **Shallower Irons:** For better crisps on your chaffles, use shallower waffle irons as they cook easier and faster.
- **Layering:** Don't fill up the waffle iron with too much batter. Work between a quarter and a half cup of total ingredients per batch for correctly done chaffles.
- **Patience:** It is a virtue even when making chaffles. For the best results, allow the chaffles to sit in the iron for 5 to 7 minutes before serving.
- **No Peeking:** 7 minutes isn't too much of a time to wait for the outcome of your chaffles, in my opinion. Opening the iron and checking on the chaffle before it is done stands you a worse chance of ruining it.
- **Crispy Cooling:** For better crisp, I find that allowing the chaffles to cool further after they are transferred to a plate aids a lot.
- **Easy Cleaning:** For the best cleanup, wet a paper towel and wipe the inner parts of the iron clean while still warm. Kindly note that the iron should be warm but not hot!
- **Brush It:** Also, use a clean toothbrush to clean between the iron's teeth for a thorough cleanup. You may also use a dry, rough sponge to clean the iron while it is still warm

CHAPTER 1:

BREAKFAST CHAFFLE RECIPES

1. Chaffles Benedict

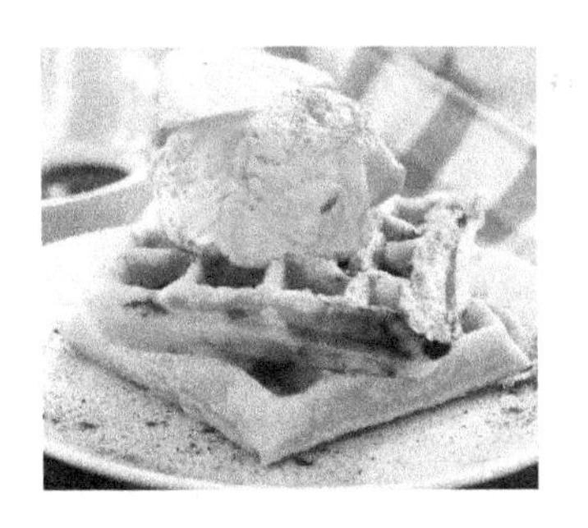

Preparation Time: 10 minutes

Difficulty level: Easy

Cooking Time: 20 minutes

Servings: 4

Ingredients: For The Chaffles:

- 12 eggs
- 1 cup cheddar cheese, shredded
- 8 slices bacon
- For the hollandaise sauce:
- 3 egg yolks
- 1 tbsp lemon juice
- 2 pinches kosher salt
- 1/4 tsp Dijon mustard or hot sauce, optional
- 1/2 cup butter, salted

Directions:

1. Preheat the waffle maker.
2. Pour water in a pan and place over medium-high heat. Take 4 eggs and beat them in a bowl. The remaining eggs are for poaching.

3. Once the waffle maker is heated up, sprinkle 1 tbsp of cheese and allow it to toast. Take 1 1/2 tbsp of the beaten eggs and place on the toasted cheese.
4. Once the egg starts cooking, add another layer of sprinkled cheese on top.
5. Close the lid. Cook for 2-3 minutes.
6. Remove the cooked chaffle and repeat the steps until you've created 8 chaffles.
7. Fry bacon and set aside for later.
8. Poach the remaining eggs.
9. To make the sauce, combine lemon juice, salt, egg yolks, and Dijon mustard or hot sauce in a bowl.
10. In a separate container, melt the butter in the microwave. Let it cool for a few minutes. Pour the melted butter over the egg yolk mixture.

11. Using an immersion blender, pulse the mixture until it becomes yellow and cloudy. Continue pulsing until the consistency becomes creamy and thick.
12. To Servings, place cooked chaffles on a plate.
13. Place a slice of bacon over each chaffle.
14. Top the bacon with poached egg and drizzle with hollandaise sauce.

Nutrition: Calories: 601 CalTotal Fat: 51 g Saturated Fat: 0 g Cholesterol: 0 mg Sodium: 0 mg Total Carbs: 1 g Fiber: 0 g Sugar: 0 g Protein: 34 g

2. Cheese-Free Breakfast Chaffle

Preparation Time: 4 minutes

Difficulty level: Easy

Cooking Time: 12 minutes **Servings:** 1

Ingredients:

- 1 egg
- ½ cup almond milk ricotta, finely shredded.
- 1 tbsp almond flour
- 2 tbsp butter

Directions:

1. Mix the egg, almond flour and ricotta in a small bowl.
2. Separate the chaffle batter into two and cook each for 4 minutes.
3. Melt the butter and pour on top of the chaffles.
4. Put them back in the pan and cook on each side for 2 minutes.

5. Remove from the pan and allow them sit for 2 minutes.
6. Enjoy while still crispy.

Nutrition: Calories: 530 CalTotal Fat: 50 g Saturated Fat: 0 g Cholesterol: 0 mg Sodium: 0 mg Total Carbs: 3 g Fiber: 0 g Sugar: 0 g Protein: 23 g

3. Breakfast Chaffle Sandwich

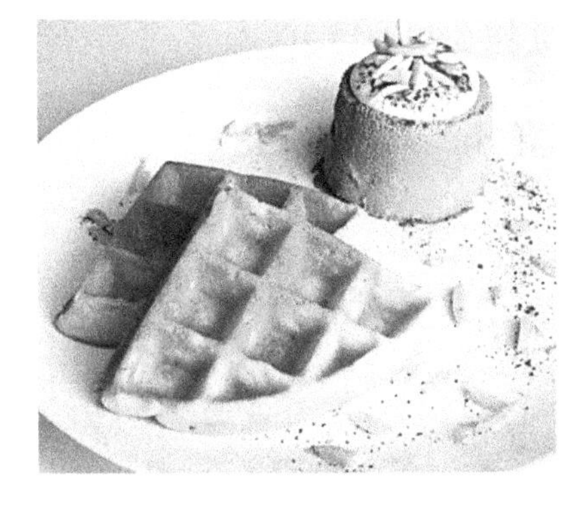

Difficulty level: Medium

Preparation Time: 5 minutes

Cooking Time: 15 minutes

Servings: 1

Ingredients:

- 1 egg
- 1/2 cup Monterey jack cheese
- 1 tbsp almond flour
- 2 tbsp butter

Directions:

1. Preheat the waffle maker for 5 minutes until it's hot.

2. Combine Monterey jack cheese, almond flour, and the egg in a bowl. Mix well.
3. Take 1/2 of the batter and pour it into the preheated waffle maker. Allow to cook for 3-4 minutes.
4. Repeat previous step for the remaining batter.
5. Melt butter on a small pan. Just like you would with French toast, add the chaffles and let each side cook for 2 minutes. To make them crispier, press down on the chaffles while they cook.
6. Remove the chaffles from the pan. Allow to cool for a few minutes. Servings.

Nutrition: Calories: 514 Cal Total Fat: 47 g Saturated Fat: 0 g Cholesterol: 0 mg

Sodium: 0 mg Total Carbs: 0 g Fiber: 0 g Sugar: 0 g Protein: 21 g

4. Ham And Jalapenos Chaffle

Preparation Time: 5 minutes

Difficulty level: Easy

Cooking Time: 9 minutes

Servings: 3

Ingredients:

- 2 lbs cheddar cheese, finely grated
- 2 large eggs
- ½ jalapeno pepper, finely grated
- 2 ounces ham steak
- 1 medium scallion
- 2 tsp coconut flour

Directions:

1. Shred the cheddar cheese using a fine grater.
2. Deseed the jalapeno and grate using the same grater.
3. Finely chop the scallion and ham.

4. Pour all the ingredients in a medium bowl and mix well.
5. Spray your waffle iron with cooking spray and heat for 3 minutes.
6. Pour 1/4 of the batter mixture into the waffle iron.
7. Cook for 3 minutes, until crispy around the edges.
8. Remove the waffles from the heat and repeat until all the batter is finished.
9. Once done, allow them to cool to room temperature and enjoy.

Nutrition: Calories: 120 Cal Total Fat: 10 g Saturated Fat: 0 g Cholesterol: 0 mg Sodium: 0 mg Total Carbs: 2 g Fiber: 0 g Sugar: 0 g Protein: 12 g

5. Crispy Zucchini Chaffle

Preparation time: 15 mins**Difficulty level:** Easy

Cooking time: 5 mins

Ingredients:

- 2 eggs 1 fresh zucchini
- 1 cup of shredded or grated cheddar cheese
- 2 pinch of salt
- 1 tablespoon of onion (chopped)
- 1 clove of garlic

Directions:

1. Start by preheating the waffle maker to medium heat. The best way to make a chaffle is to make it with layering. Start by dicing onions and mashing the garlic. Then use the grater to grate the zucchini. Then take a bowl and add 2 eggs and add the grated zucchini to the bowl.

2. Also, add the onions, salt, and garlic for extra flavor. You can also add other herbs to give your zaffle a crispy more flavor. Then sprinkle ½ cup of cheese on top of the waffle machine.
3. Add the mixture from the bowl to the waffle machine. Add the remaining cheese on top of the waffle machine and close the waffle machine. Make sure the waffle cooks for about 3 to 5 minutes until it turns golden brown.
4. By the layering method, you will achieve the perfect crisp. Take out your zucchini chaffles and serve them hot and fresh. Equipment:
5. Waffle maker
6. Grater to grate the cheese

Nutrition: Serving size 2 Calories 170 Fat 12g Carbohydrates 4g Protein 11g

6. Hot Ham Chaffles

Preparation Time: 5 minutes

Difficulty level: Medium

Cooking Time: 4 minutes

Servings: 4

Ingredients:

- ½ cup mozzarella cheese, shredded
- 1 egg
- ¼ cup ham, chopped
- ¼ tsp salt
- 2 tbsp mayonnaise
- 1 tsp Dijon mustard

Directions:

1. Preheat your waffle iron.
2. In the meantime, add the egg in a small mixing bowl and whisk.

3. Add in the ham, cheese, and salt. Mix to combine.
4. Scoop half the mixture using a spoon and pour into the hot waffle iron.
5. Close and cook for 4 minutes.
6. Remove the waffle and place on a large plate. Repeat the process with the remaining batter.
7. In a separate small bowl, add the mayo and mustard. Mix together until smooth.
8. Slice the waffles in quarters and use the mayo mixture as the dip.

Nutrition: Calories: 110 Cal Total Fat: 12 g Saturated Fat: 0 g Cholesterol: 0 mg

Sodium: 0 mg Total Carbs: 6 g Fiber: 0 g Sugar: 0 g Protein: 12 g

CHAPTER 2:

LUNCH CHAFFLE RECIPES

7. Zucchini Chaffle

Zucchini chaffle is crispy, tasty, and delicious. It is a perfect brunch meal for those on the keto diet.

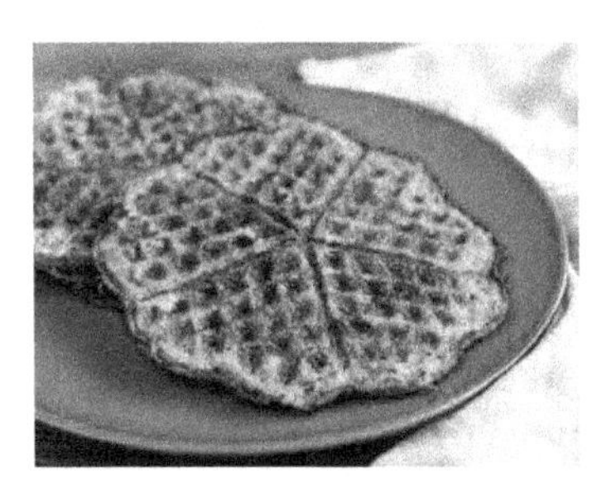

Preparation Time: 10 minutes**Difficulty level:** Easy

Cooking Time: 15 minutes **Servings**: 2

Ingredients to Use:

- 1 zucchini (grated)
- 2 eggs
- 1/2 cup of Cheddar cheese (shredded)
- 1 clove of garlic (mashed)
- 2 pinch of salt
- 1/4 cup of diced onion

Step-by-Step Directions to cook it:

1. In a bowl, add the egg, grated zucchini, onions, and garlic. Mix well.
2. Preheat the waffle-maker, add cheese and allow it to melt. Add the mixture, sprinkle more cheese, and allow to cook for 3-5 minutes or until it turns golden brown.
3. Serve hot.

Nutrition: Calorie: 170 kcal, Carbs: 4g, Fats: 10g, Protein: 13g

8. Parmesan Chicken Filled Chaffle

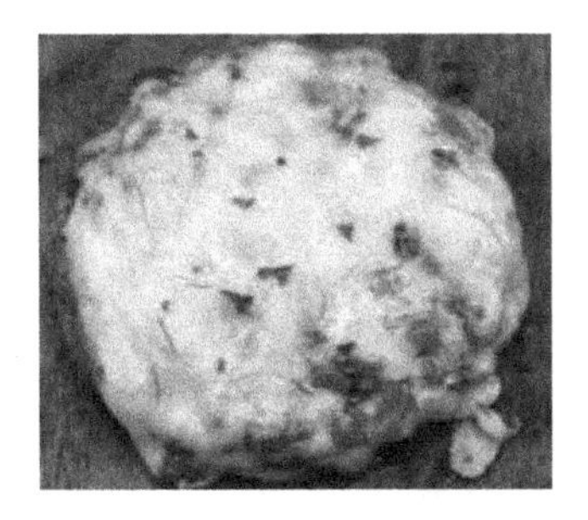

Difficulty level: Hard **Preparation Time:** 15 minutes

Cooking Time: 15 minutes **Serving:** 2

Ingredients

- 2 slices of parmesan cheese
- 1/2 cup of chicken breast (shredded)
- 1/4 cup of parmesan cheese
- 1 Tbsp of Pizza sauce
- 1 Egg
- 1/4 cup of mozzarella cheese
- 1 tsp of thick cream cheese
- 1/4 tsp of garlic powder
- 1/4 tsp of Italian seasoning

Directions

1. In a bowl, combine the shredded chicken, garlic powder, Italian seasoning, mozzarella, parmesan, cream cheese, egg, and mix until smooth.
2. Preheat your waffle-maker, sprinkle some cheese on top. Leave for seconds, pour the chicken mixture, and sprinkle some cheese. Close the waffle-maker.
3. Cook the chaffle for 3-5 minutes or until it turns golden brown. Remove and spread pizza sauce on top, add the parmesan cheese slice (make sure the chaffle is suntil hot when adding the cheese to allow it to melt).
4. Serve hot.

Nutrition : Calorie: 225kcal, Carbs: 2.1g, Fats: 8.3g, Protein: 9.3g

9. Grill Pork Chaffle Sandwich

Preparation time: 10 minutes

Servings: 2

Difficulty level: Hard

Cooking Time: 15 Minutes

Ingredients:

- 1/2 cup mozzarella, shredded
- 1 egg
- I pinch garlic powder
- PORK PATTY
- 1/2 cup pork, minutes
- 1 tbsp. green onion, diced
- 1/2 tsp Italian seasoning
- Lettuce leaves

Directions:

1. Preheat the square waffle maker and grease with

2. Mix together egg, cheese and garlic powder in a small mixing bowl.
3. Pour batter in a preheated waffle maker and close the lid.
4. Make 2 chaffles from this batter.
5. Cook chaffles for about 2-3 minutes Utes until cooked through.
6. Meanwhile, mix together pork patty ingredients in a bowl and make 1 large patty. Grill pork patty in a preheated grill for about 3-4 minutes Utes per side until cooked through.
7. Arrange pork patty between two chaffles with lettuce leaves. Cut sandwich to make a triangular sandwich. Enjoy!

Nutrition: Protein: 48% 85 kcal Fat: 48% 86 kcal Carbohydrates: 4% 7 kcal

CHAPTER 3:

DINNER CHAFFLES

10. Jalapeno Chicken Popper Chaffles

Jalapeno chicken popper is a great meal for anyone on a keto diet. It tastes better with sauce or toppings.

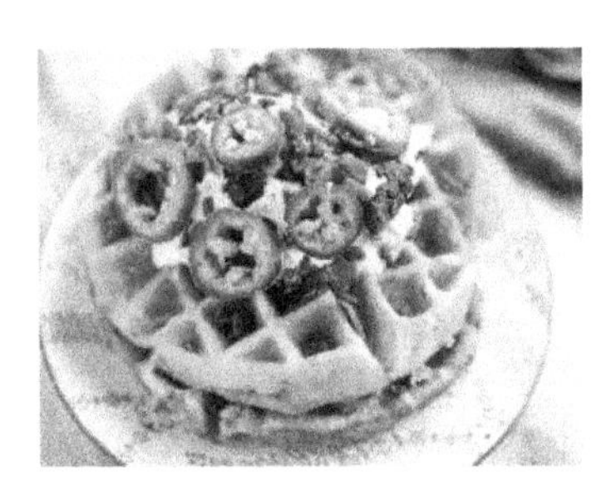

Difficulty: Hard **Servings:** 2 **Preparatio Time:** 5 minutes

Cooking Time: 15minutes

Ingredients:

- 1/2 cup of chicken (shredded)

- 1/4 cup of mozzarella cheese
- 1/4 tsp of garlic powder
- 1/4 cup of parmesan cheese
- 1/4 tsp of onion powder
- 1 fresh jalapeno (diced)
- 1 egg - 1 tsp of cream cheese

Step-by-Step Directions to cook it:

1. Preheat the waffle-maker.
2. In a bowl, add all the ingredients and mix thoroughly.
3. Sprinkle cheese on the waffle-maker and heat for 20 seconds. Pour the mixture on top and allow it to cook for 3-4 minutes. Serve with any sauce or toppings of choice

Nutrition: Calorie: 231.4kcal, Carbs: 4.5g, Fats: 10.6g, Protein: 19.2g

11. Chicken Mozzarella Chaffle

Difficulty level: Hard

Preparation Time: 5 minutes

Cooking time: 10 minutes **Servings:** 2

Ingredients:

- Chicken: 1 cup
- Egg: 2
- Mozzarella cheese: 1 cup and 4 tbsp
- Tomato sauce: 6 tbsp
- Basil: ½ tsp
- Garlic: ½ tbsp
- Butter: 1 tsp

Direction:

1. In a pan, add butter and include small pieces of chicken to it
2. Stir for two minutes and then add garlic and basil

3. Set aside the cooked chicken
4. Preheat the mini waffle maker if needed
5. Mix cooked chicken, eggs, and 1 cup mozzarella cheese properly
6. Spread it to the mini waffle maker thoroughly
7. Cook for 4 minutes or till it turns crispy and then remove it from the waffle maker Make as many mini chaffles as you can
8. Now in a baking tray, line these mini chaffles and top with the tomato sauce and grated mozzarella cheese
9. Put the tray in the oven at 400 degrees until the cheese melts Serve hot

Nutrition: Calories: 188 | Carbohydrates: 1.3g | Fat: 11.1g | Protein: 18.7g | Cholesterol: 173mg

12. Crunchy Keto Cinnamon Chaffle

Preparation Time: 5 minutes **Difficulty level:** Hard

Cooking Time: 10 minutes Servings: 2

Ingredients

- 1 tablespoon almond flour
- 1 egg
- 1 teaspoon of vanilla
- Cinnamon 1 shake
- 1 teaspoon baking powder
- 1 cup mozzarella cheese

Directions

1. Mix the egg and vanilla extract in a bowl.
2. Mix powder, almond flour and cinnamon with baking.
3. Finally, add the cheese in the mozzarella and coat with the mixture evenly. Spray oil on your waffle

maker and let it heat up to its maximum setting. Cook the waffle, test it every 5 minutes until it becomes golden and crunchy. A tip: make sure you put half of the batter in it. It can overflow the waffle maker, rendering it a sloppy operation. I suggest you put down a silpat mat to make it easy to clean.

4. With butter and your favorite low-carb syrup, take it out carefully.

Nutrition: Calories 450, Calories from Fat 141, Fat 15.7g, sodium 209mg, potassium 128mg, carbohydrates 9.9g, Fiber 2.9g, sugar 0.9g, Protein 11.5g, vitamin a 345iu, calcium 175mg, iron 1.8mg

13.Garlic Chicken Chaffle

Difficulty level: Hard

Preparation Time: 10 minutes

Cooking Time: 25 minutes

Serving: 2

Ingredients:

- Chicken: 3-4 pieces
- Lemon juice: ½ tbsp
- Garlic: 1 clove
- Kewpie mayo: 2 tbsp
- Egg: 1
- Mozzarella cheese: ½ cup
- Salt: As per your taste

Direction:

1. In a pot, cook the chicken by adding one cup of water to it with salt and bring to boil

2. Close the lid of the pot and cook for 15-20 minutes
3. When done, remove from stove and shred the chicken pieces leaving the bones behind; discard the bones
4. Grate garlic finely into pieces
5. Beat the egg in the mixing bowl, add garlic, lemon juice, Kewpie mayo, and 1/8 cup of cheese
6. Preheat the waffle maker if needed and grease it
7. Add the mixture to the waffle maker and cook for 4-5 minutes or until it is done
8. Remove the chaffles from the pan and preheat the oven
9. In the meanwhile, set the chaffles on a baking tray and spread the chicken on them
10. After that, sprinkle the remaining cheese on the chaffles

11. Put the tray in the oven and heat till the cheese melts
12. Serve hot
13. Make as many chaffles as you like

Nutrition : Calorie: 198kcal, Carbs: 3 1g, Fats: 8.4g, Protein: 6g

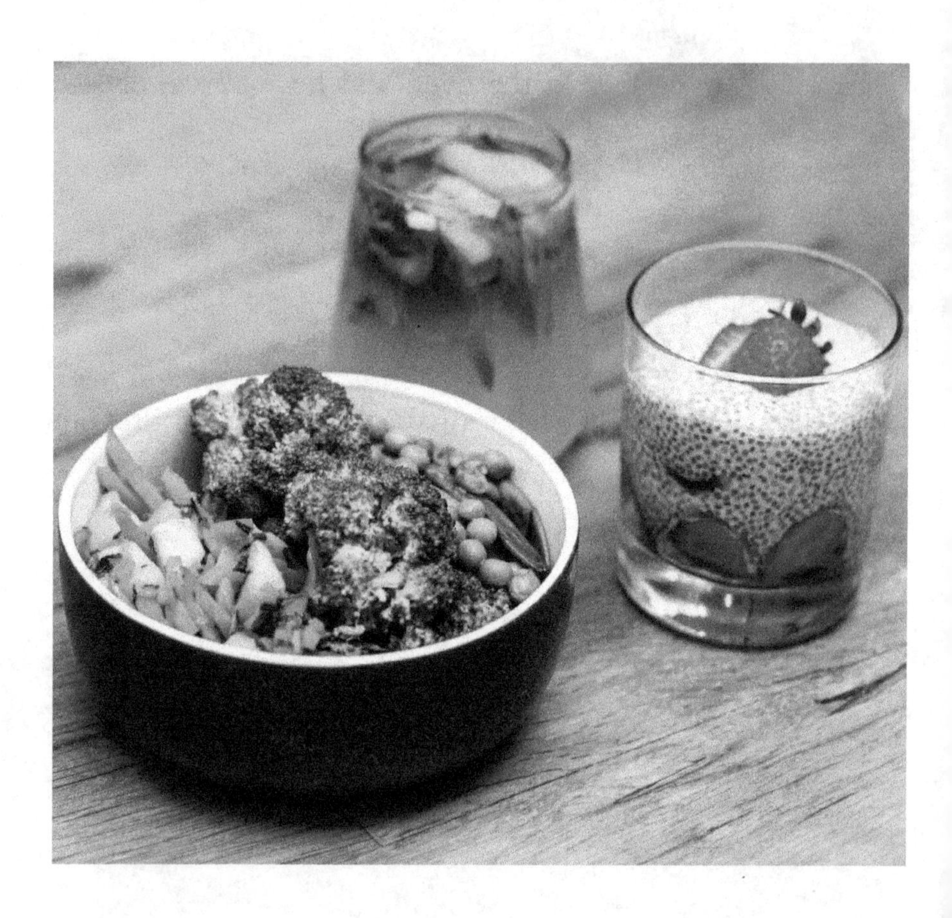

CHAPTER 4:

CHAFFLE CAKE & SANDWICH RECIPES

14. Salmon & Cheese Sandwich Chaffles

Preparation time: 6 minutes

Difficulty level: Hard

Servings: 4

Cooking Time: 24 Minutes

Ingredients:

- Chaffles
- 2 organic eggs

- ½ ounce butter, melted
- 1 cup mozzarella cheese, shredded
- 2 tablespoons almond flour
- Pinch of salt
- Filling
- ½ cup smoked salmon
- 1/3 cup avocado, peeled, pitted, and sliced
- 2 tablespoons feta cheese, crumbled

Directions:

1. Preheat a mini waffle iron and then grease it.
2. For chaffles: In a medium bowl, put all ingredients and with a fork, mix until well combined.
3. Place ¼ of the mixture into preheated waffle iron and cook for about 5–6 minutes.
4. Repeat with the remaining mixture.

5. Serve each chaffle with filling ingredients.

Nutrition: Calories 169 Net Carbs 1.2 g

Total Fat 13.g Saturated Fat 5 g

Cholesterol 101 mg Sodium 319 mg

Total Carbs 2.8 g Fiber 1.6 g Sugar 0.6 g Protein 8.9 g

15. Chicken Sandwich Chaffles

Preparation time: 6 minutes .

Servings: 2

Difficulty level: Hard

Cooking Time: 8 Minutes

Ingredients:

- Chaffles
- 1 large organic egg, beaten
- ½ cup cheddar cheese, shredded
- Pinch of salt and ground black pepper
- Filling
- 1 (6-ounce) cooked chicken breast, halved
- 2 lettuce leaves ¼ of small onion, sliced
- 1 small tomato, sliced

Directions:

1. Preheat a mini waffle iron and then grease it.

2. For chaffles: In a medium bowl, put all ingredients and with a fork, mix until well combined. Place half of the mixture into preheated waffle iron and cook for about 3–4 minutes.
3. Repeat with the remaining mixture.
4. Serve each chaffle with filling ingredients.

Nutrition: Calories 2 Net Carbs 2.5 g Total Fat 14.1 g Saturated Fat 6.8 g Cholesterol 177 mg Sodium 334 mg Total Carbs 3.3 g Fiber 0.8 g Sugar 2 g Protein 28.7 g

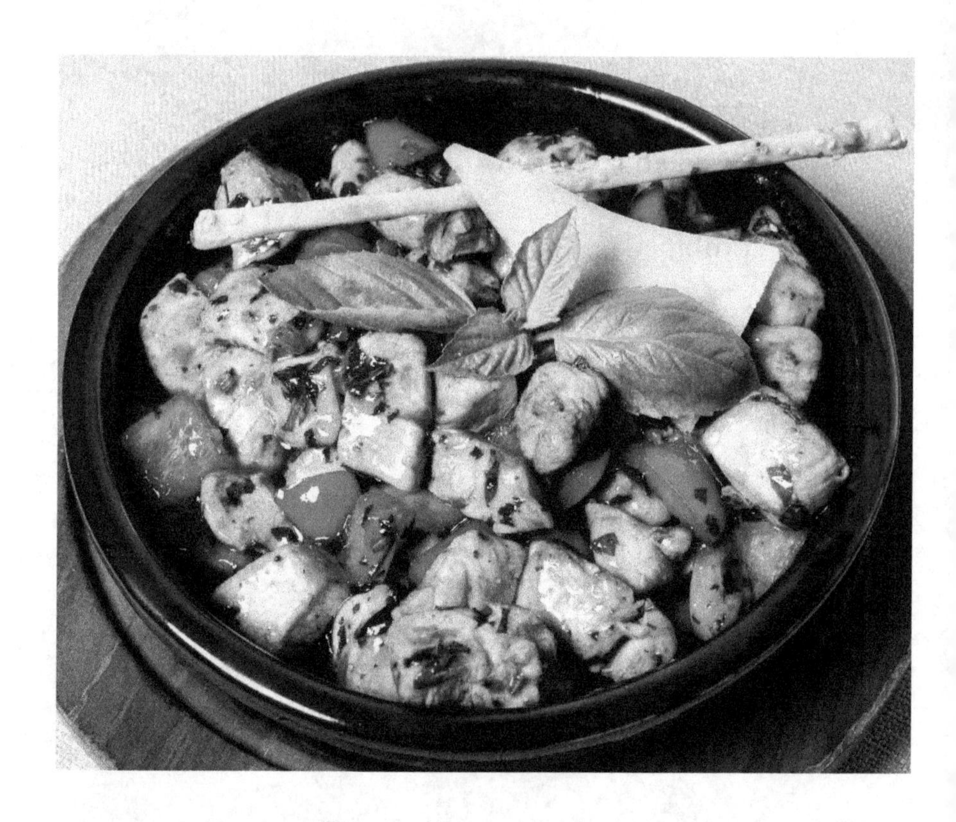

CHAPTER 5:

VEGETARIAN CHAFFLE RECIPES

16. Cinnamon Roll Keto Chaffles

Preparation time: 10 minutes **Difficulty level:** Hard

Cooking Time: 10 Minutes

Servings: 2

Ingredients:

- Cinnamon Roll Chaffle
- 1/2 cup mozzarella cheese
- 1 tablespoon almond flour

- 1/4 tsp baking powder
- 1 egg
- 1 tsp cinnamon
- 1 tsp Granulated Swerve
- Cinnamon roll swirl
- 1 tbsp butter
- 1 tsp cinnamon
- 2 tsp confectioners swerve
- Keto Cinnamon Roll Glaze
- 1 tablespoon butter
- 1 tablespoon cream cheese
- 1/4 tsp vanilla extract
- 2 tsp swerve confectioners

Directions:

1. Plug in your Mini Dash Waffle maker and let it heat up.

2. In a small bowl mix the mozzarella cheese, almond flour, baking powder, egg, 1 teaspoon cinnamon, and 1 teaspoon swerve granulated and set aside.
3. In another small bowl, add a tablespoon of butter, 1 teaspoon cinnamon, and 2 teaspoons of swerve confectioners' sweetener.
4. Microwave for 15 seconds and mix well.
5. Spray the waffle maker with nonstick spray and add 1/3 of the batter to your waffle maker. Swirl in 1/3 of the cinnamon, swerve, and butter mixture onto the top of it. Close the waffle maker and let cook for 3-4 minutes.
6. When the first cinnamon roll chaffle is done, make the second and then make the third.
7. While the third chaffle is cooking place 1 tablespoon butter and 1 tablespoon of cream

cheese in a small bowl. Heat in the microwave for 10-15 seconds. Start at 10, and if the cream cheese is not soft enough to mix with the butter heat for an additional 5 seconds.

8. Add the vanilla extract, and the swerve confectioner's sweetener to the butter and cream cheese and mix well using a whisk.
9. Drizzle keto cream cheese glaze on top of chaffle.

Nutrition: Caloris:180kcal;Carbohydrates:3g;Protein:7g;Fat:16g;SaturatedFat:9g;Cholesterol:95mg;Sodium:221mg;Potassium: 77mg;Fiber: 1g;Sugar: 1g;Vitamin A: 505IU;Calcium: 148mg;Iron: 1mg

CHAPTER 6:

BASIC CHAFFLES RECIPES

17.Light & Crispy Bagel Chaffle Chips

Preparation time: 5 minutes

Difficulty level: EASY

Cooking time: 5 minutes **Servings:** 4

Ingredients:

- 3 tbsp. parmesan cheese 1 tsp oil for grease
- 1 tsp bagel seasoning Salt and pepper to taste

Directions:

Preheat the waffle maker. Add the parmesan cheese in the pan and melt it well. Now pour the melted parmesan cheese over the waffle maker and sprinkle bagel seasoning over the cheese. Cook the mixture for about 2 to 3 minutes without closing the lid. Let it settle or turn crispy for 2 minutes then remove and serve the crispy chis crunch.

Nutrition: Calories 320 Carbohydrates 2.9 g Protein 21.5 g Fat 24.3g

18. Simple Brownie Chaffle

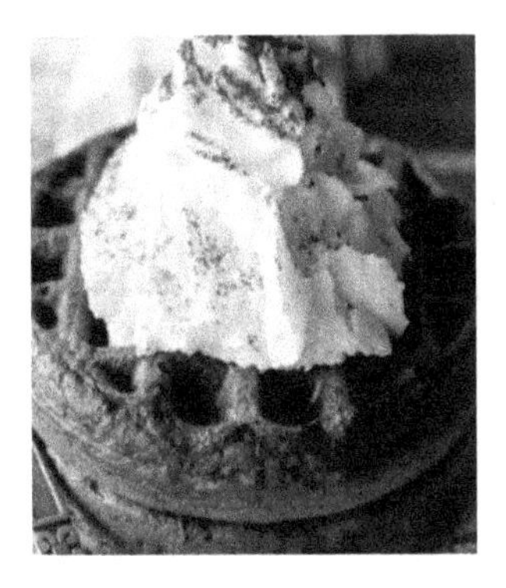

Difficulty level: EASY

Preparation time: 5 minutes

Cooking time: 3 minutes **Servings:** 2

If you love brownies, then you should try this brownie Chaffle recipe which is very easy to make and is ready in few minutes.

Ingredients

- 1 Egg Whisked
- 1/3 cup Mozzarella Cheese Shredded
- 1 ½ tbsp Cocoa Powder Dutch Processed
- 1 tbsp Almond Flour

- 1 tbsp Monk fruit Sweetener
- 1/4 tsp Vanilla extract
- 1/4 tsp Baking Powder
- Pinch of Salt
- 2 tsp Heavy Cream

Directions

1. First step as always is to preheat your mini waffle iron.
2. Next, whisk the egg. Add the dry ingredients. Then add the cheese in a bowl. Then you Pour 1/3 of the batter on the waffle iron. Allow to cook for 3 minutes or until steam stops coming out of the waffle iron.
3. Serve with your favorite low carb toppings.

Nutrition: Calories 320 Carbohydrates 2.9 g 21.5 g Fat 24.3g

CHAPTER 7:

SWEET CHAFFLES RECIPES

19. Pumpkin & Psyllium Husk Chaffles

Preparation time: 8 minutes

Difficulty level: Easy

Cooking Time: 16 Minutes

Servings: 2

Ingredients:

- 2 organic eggs
- ½ cup mozzarella cheese, shredded
- 1 tablespoon homemade pumpkin puree
- 2 teaspoons Erythritol

- ½ teaspoon psyllium husk powder
- 1/3 teaspoon ground cinnamon
- Pinch of salt
- ½ teaspoon organic vanilla extract

Directions:

1. Preheat a mini waffle iron and then grease it. In a bowl, place all ingredients and beat until well combined.
2. Place ¼ of the mixture into preheated waffle iron and cook for about 4 minutes or until golden brown. Repeat with the remaining mixture.
3. Serve warm.

Nutrition: Calories: 4et Carb: 0.6gFat: 2.8gSaturated Fat: 1.1gCarbohydrates: 0.8gDietary Fiber: 0.2g Sugar: 0.4gProtein: 3.9g

20. Pumpkin Chaffles

Preparation time: 5 minutes

Difficulty level: Easy

Cooking Time: 12 Minutes **Servings:** 3

Ingredients:

- 1 organic egg, beaten
- ½ cup Mozzarella cheese, shredded
- 1½ tablespoon homemade pumpkin puree
- ½ teaspoon Erythritol
- ½ teaspoon organic vanilla extract
- ¼ teaspoon pumpkin pie spice

Directions:

1. Preheat a mini waffle iron and then grease it. In a bowl, place all the ingredients and beat until well combined.

2. Place ¼ of the mixture into preheated waffle iron and cook for about 4-6 minutes or until golden brown. Repeat with the remaining mixture. Serve warm.

Nutrition: Calories: 59Net Carb: 1.2gFat: 3.5gSaturated Fat: 1.5gCarbohydrates: 1.Dietary Fiber: 0.4g Sugar: 0.7gProtein: 4.9g

21. Raspberry Chaffles

Preparation time: 5 minutes **Difficulty level:** Easy

cooking Time: 5 Minutes **Servings:** 5

Ingredients:

- 4 Tbsp almond flour
- 4 large eggs
- 2⅓ cup shredded mozzarella cheese
- 1 tsp vanilla extract
- 1 Tbsp erythritol sweetener
- 1½ tsp baking powder
- ½ cup raspberries

Directions:

1. Turn on waffle maker to heat and oil it with cooking spray.
2. Mix almond flour, sweetener, and baking powder in a bowl.

3. Add cheese, eggs, and vanilla extract, and mix until well-combined.
4. Add 1 portion of batter to waffle maker and spread it evenly. Close and cook for 3-minutes, or until golden.
5. Repeat until remaining batter is used.
6. Serve with raspberries.

Nutrition: Carbs: 5 g ;Fat: 11 g ;Protein: 24 g ;Calories: 300

22. Mozzarella & Butter Chaffles

Preparation time: 5 minutes **Difficulty level:** Easy

Cooking Time: 8 Minutes

Servings: 2

Ingredients:

- 1 large organic egg, beaten
- ¾ cup Mozzarella cheese, shredded
- ½ tablespoon unsalted butter, melted
- 2 tablespoons blanched almond flour
- 2 tablespoons Erythritol
- ½ teaspoon ground cinnamon
- ½ teaspoon Psyllium husk powder
- ¼ teaspoon organic baking powder
- ½ teaspoon organic vanilla extract

Directions:

1. Preheat a waffle iron and then grease it.

2. In a medium bowl, place all ingredients and with a fork, mix until well combined.
3. Place half of the mixture into preheated waffle iron and cook for about 5 minutes or until golden brown.
4. Repeat with the remaining mixture.
5. Serve warm.

Nutrition: Calories: 140Net Carb: 1.9gFat: 10.Saturated Fat: 4gCarbohydrates: 3gDietary Fiber: 1.1g Sugar: 0.3gProtein: 7.8g

23. Cream Cheese Chaffles

Preparation time: 5 minutes

Difficulty level: Easy

Cooking Time: 8 Minutes

Servings: 2

Ingredients:

- 2 teaspoons coconut flour
- 3 teaspoons Erythritol
- ¼ teaspoon organic baking powder
- 1 organic egg, beaten
- 1 ounce cream cheese, softened
- ½ teaspoon organic vanilla extract

Directions:

6. Preheat a mini waffle iron and then grease it.
7. In a bowl, place flour, Erythritol and baking powder and mix well.

8. Add the egg, cream cheese and vanilla extract and beat until well combined.
9. Place half of the mixture into preheated waffle iron and cook for about 3-minutes or until golden brown.
10. Repeat with the remaining mixture.
11. Serve warm.

Nutrition: Calories: 95Net Carb: 1.6gFat: 4gSaturated Fat: 4gCarbohydrates: 2.6gDietary Fiber: 1g Sugar: 0.3gProtein: 4.2g

CHAPTER 8:

DESSERT CHAFFLES

24. Sweet Vanilla Chocolate Chaffle

Preparation time: 10 minutes

Difficulty level: Hard

Cooking Time: 10 Minutes

Servings: 2

Ingredients:

- 1 egg, lightly beaten
- 1/4 tsp cinnamon
- 1/2 tsp vanilla
- 1 tbsp Swerve

- 2 tsp unsweetened cocoa powder
- 1 tbsp coconut flour
- 2 oz cream cheese, softened

Directions:

1. Add all ingredients into the small bowl and mix until well combined.
2. Spray waffle maker with cooking spray.
3. Pour batter in the hot waffle maker and cook until golden brown.
4. Serve and enjoy.

Nutrition: Calories 312Fat 24 carbohydrates 11.5 sugar 0.8 protein 11.6 cholesterol 226 mg

25. Maple Syrup & Vanilla Chaffle

Preparation time: 6 minutes

Cooking Time: 12 Minutes

Difficulty level: Hard

Servings: 2

Ingredients:

- 1 egg, beaten
- ¼ cup mozzarella cheese, shredded
- 1 oz. cream cheese
- 1 teaspoon vanilla
- 1 tablespoon keto maple syrup
- 1 teaspoon sweetener
- 1 teaspoon baking powder
- 4 tablespoons almond flour

Directions:

1. Preheat your waffle maker.

2. Add all the ingredients to a bowl.
3. Mix well.
4. Pour some of the batter into the waffle maker.
5. Cover and cook for 4 minutes.
6. Transfer chaffle to a plate and let cool for 2 minutes.
7. Repeat the same process with the remaining mixture.

Nutrition: Calories 146 Total Fat 9.5g Saturated Fat 4.3g Cholesterol 99mg Potassium 322mg Sodium 99mg Total Carbohydrate 10.6g Dietary Fiber 0.9g Protein 5.6g Total Sugars 6.4g

26. Cheese Garlic Chaffle

Preparation time: 10 minutes

Difficulty level: Easy

Cooking Time: 8 Minutes

Servings: 2

Ingredients:

- Chaffle
- 1 egg
- 1 teaspoon cream cheese
- ½ cup mozzarella cheese, shredded
- ½ teaspoon garlic powder
- 1 teaspoon Italian seasoning
- Topping
- 1 tablespoon butter
- ½ teaspoon garlic powder
- ½ teaspoon Italian seasoning

- 2 tablespoon mozzarella cheese, shredded

Directions:

1. Plug in your waffle maker to preheat.
2. Preheat your oven to 350 degrees F.
3. In a bowl, combine all the chaffle ingredients.
4. Cook in the waffle maker for minutes per chaffle.
5. Transfer to a baking pan.
6. Spread butter on top of each chaffle.
7. Sprinkle garlic powder and Italian seasoning on top.
8. Top with mozzarella cheese.
9. Bake until the cheese has melted.

Nutrition: Calories141 Total Fat 13 g Saturated Fat 8 g Cholesterol 115.8 mg Sodium 255.8 mg Potassium 350 mg Total Carbohydrate 2.6g Dietary Fiber 0.7g

27. Carrot Cake Chaffle

Difficulty level: Easy **Preparation Time:** 10 minutes

Cooking Time: 18 minutes **Servings:** 10 (6 mini chaffles)

Ingredients:

- 1 tbsp toasted pecans (chopped)
- 2 tbsp granulated swerve
- 1 tsp pumpkin spice 1 tsp baking powder
- ½ shredded carrots 2 tbsp butter (melted)
- 1 tsp cinnamon 1 tsp vanilla extract (optional)
- 2 tbsp heavy whipping cream
- ¾ cup almond flour 1 egg (beaten)
- Butter cream cheese frosting:
- ½ cup cream cheese (softened)
- ¼ cup butter (softened)
- ½ tsp vanilla extract
- ¼ cup granulated swerve

Directions:

1. Plug the chaffle maker to preheat it and spray it with a non-stick cooking spray.
2. In a mixing bowl, combine the almond flour, cinnamon, carrot, pumpkin spice and swerve.
3. In another mixing bowl, whisk together the eggs, butter, heavy whipping cream, and vanilla extract.
4. Pour the flour mixture into the egg mixture and mix until you form a smooth batter.
5. Fold in the chopped pecans.
6. Close the waffle maker and cook for about 3 minutes or according to your waffle maker's settings.
7. After the cooking cycle, use a plastic or silicone utensil to remove the chaffle from the waffle maker.
8. Repeat steps 6 to 8 until you have cooked all the batter into chaffless.

9. For the frosting, combine the cream cheese and cutter int a mixer and mix until well combined.
10. Add the swerve and vanilla extract and slowly until the sweetener is well incorporated. Mix on high until the frosting is fluffy.
11. Place one chaffle on a flat surface and spread some cream frosting over it. Layer another chaffle over the first one a spread some cream over it too.
12. Repeat step 12 until you have assembled all the chaffless into a cake.
13. Cut and serve.

Nutrition: Servings: 10 Amount per serving Calories 181 % Daily Value* Total Fat 17.4g 22% Saturated Fat 8.1g 41% Cholesterol 52mg 17% Sodium 93mg 4% Total Carbohydrate 4.5g 2% Dietary Fiber 1.2g 4% Total Sugars 0.6g Protein 3.5g Vitamin D 8mcg 39% Calcium 61mg 5% Iron 1mg 4% Potassium 91mg 2%

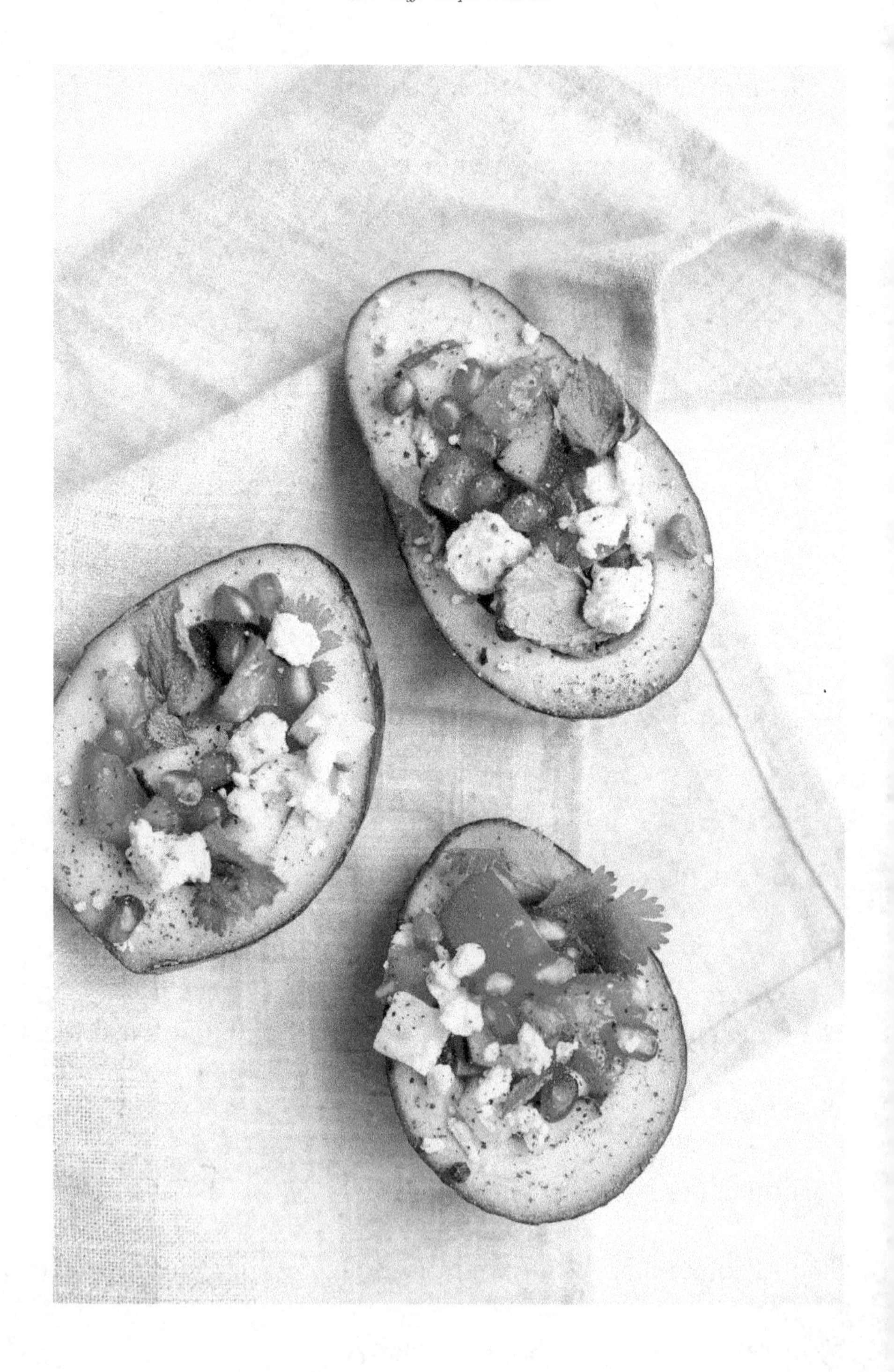

CHAPTER 9:

SAVORY CHAFFLES RECIPES

28. Garlic And Spinach Chaffles

Preparation time: 6 minutes

Cooking Time: 5 minutes

Difficulty level: Medium **Servings:** 2

Ingredients:

- 1 cup egg whites
- 1 tsp. Italian spice
- 2 tsps. coconut flour

- ½ tsp. Vanilla
- 1 tsp. baking powder
- 1 tsp. baking soda
- 1 cup mozzarella cheese, grated
- 1/2 tsp. garlic powder
- 1 cup chopped spinach

Directions:

1. Switch on your square waffle maker. Spray with non-stick spray.
2. Beat egg whites with beater, until fluffy and white.
3. Add pumpkin puree, pumpkin pie spice, coconut flour in egg whites and beat again.
4. Stir in the cheese, powder, garlic powder, baking soda, and powder.
5. Sprinkle chopped spinach on a waffle maker Pour the batter in waffle maker over chopped spinach

6. Close the maker and cook for about 4-5 minutes Utes. Remove chaffles from the maker.
7. Serve hot and enjoy!

Nutrition: Protein: 52% 88 kcal Fat: 41% 69 kcal Carbohydrates: 7% 12 kcal

29. Zucchini Chaffles With Peanut Butter

Servings:2

Preparation time: 6 minutes

Difficulty level: Easy

Cooking Time: 5 Minutes

Ingredients:

- 1 cup zucchini grated
- 1 egg beaten
- 1/2 cup shredded parmesan cheese
- 1/4 cup shredded mozzarella cheese
- 1 tsp dried basil
- 1/2 tsp. salt 1/2 tsp. black pepper
- 2 tbsps. peanut butter for topping

Directions:

1. Sprinkle salt over zucchini and let it sit for minutes Utes.

2. Squeeze out water from zucchini.
3. Beat egg with zucchini, basil. salt mozzarella cheese, and pepper.
4. Sprinkle ½ of the parmesan cheese over preheated waffle maker and pour zucchini batter over it. Sprinkle the remaining cheese over it.
5. Close the lid. Cook zucchini chaffles for about 4-8 minutes Utes.
6. Remove chaffles from the maker and repeat with the remaining batter.
7. Serve with peanut butter on top and enjoy!

Nutrition: Protein: 52% 88 kcal Fat: 41% 69 kcal Carbohydrates: 7% 12 kcal

30. Breakfast Chaffle

Preparation time: 6 minutes

Difficulty: Easy **Cooking Time:** 5 Minutes **Servings:** 2

Ingredients:

- 2 eggs
- ½ cup shredded mozzarella cheese
- For the toppings: 2 ham slices 1 fried egg

Directions:

1. Mix eggs and cheese in a small bowl.
2. Turn on waffle maker to heat and oil it with cooking spray. Pour half of the batter into the waffle maker. Cook for 2-minutes, remove, and repeat with remaining batter.
3. Place egg and ham between two chaffles to make a sandwich.

Nutrition: Carbs: 1 g ;Fat: 8 g ;Protein: 9 g ;Calories: 115

31. Chaffle Cuban Sandwich

Preparation time: 5 minutes **Difficulty level:** Easy

Cooking Time: 10 Minutes **Servings:** 2

Ingredients:

- 1 large egg 1 Tbsp almond flour
- 1 Tbsp full-fat Greek yogurt
- ⅛ tsp baking powder
- ¼ cup shredded Swiss cheese
- For the Filling:
- 3 oz roast pork 2 oz deli ham
- 1 slice Swiss cheese
- 3-5 sliced pickle chips
- ½ Tbsp Dijon mustard

Directions:

1. Turn on waffle maker to heat and oil it with cooking spray.

2. Beat egg, yogurt, almond flour, and baking powder in a bowl.
3. Sprinkle ¼ Swiss cheese on hot waffle maker. Top with half of the egg mixture, then add ¼ of the cheese on top. Close and cook for 5 minutes, until golden brown and crispy.
4. Repeat with remaining batter.
5. Layer pork, ham, and cheese slice in a small microwaveable bowl. Microwave for seconds, until cheese melts.
6. Spread the inside of chaffle with mustard and top with pickles. Invert bowl onto chaffle top so that cheese is touching pickles. Place bottom chaffle onto pork and serve.

Nutrition: Carbs: 4 g ;Fat: 46 g ;Protein: 33 g ;Calories: 522

32. Cauliflower & Italian Seasoning Chaffles

Preparation time: 10 minutes

Difficulty level: Easy

Cooking Time: 20 Minutes

Servings: 2

Ingredients:

- 1 cup cauliflower rice
- ¼ teaspoon garlic powder
- ½ teaspoon Italian seasoning
- Salt and freshly ground black pepper, to taste
- ½ cup Mexican blend cheese, shredded
- 1 organic egg, beaten
- ½ cup Parmesan cheese, shredded

Directions:

1. Preheat a mini waffle iron and then grease it.

2. In a blender, add all the ingredients except Parmesan cheese and pulse until well combined.
3. Place 1½ tablespoon of the Parmesan cheese in the bottom of preheated waffle iron.
4. Place ¼ of the egg mixture over cheese and sprinkle with the ½ tablespoon of the Parmesan cheese.
5. Cook for about 4-minutes or until golden brown.
6. Repeat with the remaining mixture and Parmesan cheese.
7. Serve warm.

Nutrition: Calories: 127Net Carb: 2gFat: 9gSaturated Fat: 5.3gCarbohydrates: 2.7gDietary Fiber: 0.7g Sugar: 1.5gProtein: 9.2g

33. Taco Chaffle Shell

Preparation time: 5 minutes **Difficulty level:** Easy

Cooking Time: 8 Minutes

Servings: 2

Ingredients:

- 1 egg white
- ¼ cup shredded Monterey jack cheese
- ¼ cup shredded sharp cheddar cheese
- ¾ tsp water
- 1 tsp coconut flour
- ¼ tsp baking powder
- ⅛ tsp chili powder
- Pinch of salt

Directions:

1. Turn on waffle maker to heat and oil it with cooking spray.

2. Mix all components in a bowl.
3. Spoon half of the batter on the waffle maker and cook for 4 minutes.
4. Remove chaffle and set aside. Repeat for remaining chaffle batter.
5. Turn over a muffin pan and set chaffle between the cups to form a shell. Allow to set for 2-4 minutes.
6. Remove and serve with your favorite taco recipe.

Nutrition: Carbs: 4 g ;Fat: 19 g ;Protein: 18 g ;Calories: 258

34. Garlic Powder Chaffles

Preparation time: 6 minutes

Difficulty level: Easy

Cooking Time: 8 Minutes

Servings: 2

Ingredients:

- 1 organic egg, beaten
- ½ cup Monterrey Jack cheese, shredded
- 1 teaspoon coconut flour
- Pinch of garlic powder

Directions:

1. Preheat a mini waffle iron and then grease it.
2. In a bowl, place all the ingredients and beat until well combined.
3. Place half of the mixture into preheated waffle iron and cook for about 4 minutes or until golden brown.
4. Repeat with the remaining mixture.

5. Serve warm.

Nutrition: Calories: 147Net Carb: 1.Fat: 11.3gSaturated Fat: 6.8gCarbohydrates: 2.1gDietary Fiber: 0.5g Sugar: 0.2gProtein: 9g

CHAPTER 10:

FESTIVE CHAFFLE RECIPES

35. Maple Chaffle

Preparation time: 10 minutes Difficulty level: Medium

Cooking Time: 15 Minutes

Servings: 2

Ingredients:

- 1 egg, lightly beaten
- 2 egg whites
- 1/2 tsp maple extract

- 2 tsp Swerve
- 1/2 tsp baking powder, gluten-free
- 2 tbsp almond milk
- 2 tbsp coconut flour

Directions:

1. Preheat your waffle maker.
2. In a bowl, whip egg whites until stiff peaks form.
3. Stir in maple extract, Swerve, baking powder, almond milk, coconut flour, and egg.
4. Spray waffle maker with cooking spray.
5. Pour half batter in the hot waffle maker and cook for 3-minutes or until golden brown. Repeat with the remaining batter.
6. Serve and enjoy.

Nutrition: Calories 122Fat 6.6 carbohydrates 9 sugar 1 protein 7 cholesterol 82 mg

36. Choco Chip Pumpkin Chaffle

Preparation time: 10 minutes

Difficulty level: Medium

Cooking Time: 15 Minutes

Servings: 2

Ingredients:

- 1 egg, lightly beaten
- 1 tbsp almond flour
- 1 tbsp unsweetened chocolate chips
- 1/4 tsp pumpkin pie spice
- 2 tbsp Swerve
- 1 tbsp pumpkin puree
- 1/2 cup mozzarella cheese, shredded

Directions:

1. Preheat your waffle maker.
2. In a small bowl, mix egg and pumpkin puree.

3. Add pumpkin pie spice, Swerve, almond flour, and cheese and mix well.
4. Stir in chocolate chips.
5. Spray waffle maker with cooking spray.
6. Pour half batter in the hot waffle maker and cook for 4 minutes. Repeat with the remaining batter.
7. Serve and enjoy.

Nutrition: Calories 130Fat 9.2 carbohydrates 5.9 sugar 0.6 protein 6.6 cholesterol mg

37. Pizza Flavored Chaffle

Preparation time: 6 minutes

Difficulty level: Medium

Cooking Time: 12 Minutes

Servings: 2

Ingredients:

- 1 egg, beaten
- ½ cup cheddar cheese, shredded
- 2 tablespoons pepperoni, chopped
- 1 tablespoon keto marinara sauce
- 4 tablespoons almond flour
- 1 teaspoon baking powder
- ½ teaspoon dried Italian seasoning
- Parmesan cheese, grated

Directions:

1. Preheat your waffle maker.

2. In a bowl, mix the egg, cheddar cheese, pepperoni, marinara sauce, almond flour, baking powder and Italian seasoning.
3. Add the mixture to the waffle maker.
4. Close the device and cook for minutes.
5. Open it and transfer chaffle to a plate.
6. Let cool for 2 minutes.
7. Repeat the steps with the remaining batter.
8. Top with the grated Parmesan and serve.

Nutrition: Calories 17 Total Fat 14.3g Saturated Fat 7.5g Cholesterol 118mg Sodium 300mg Potassium 326mg Total Carbohydrate 1.8g Dietary Fiber 0.1g Protein 11.1g Total Sugars 0.4g

38. Sausage & Pepperoni Chaffle Sandwich

Preparation time: 8 minutes

Difficulty level: Medium

Cooking Time: 10 Minutes

Servings: 2

Ingredients:

- Cooking spray
- 2 cervelat sausage, sliced into rounds
- 12 pieces pepperoni
- 6 mushroom slices
- 4 teaspoons mayonnaise
- 4 big white onion rings
- 4 basic chaffles

Directions:

1. Spray your skillet with oil.
2. Place over medium heat.

3. Cook the sausage until brown on both sides.
4. Transfer on a plate.
5. Cook the pepperoni and mushrooms for 2 minutes.
6. Spread mayo on top of the chaffle.
7. Top with the sausage, pepperoni, mushrooms and onion rings.
8. Top with another chaffle.

Nutrition: Calories 373 Total Fat 24.4g Saturated Fat 6g Cholesterol 27mg Sodium 717mg Potassium 105mg Total Carbohydrate 28g Dietary Fiber 1.1g Protein 8.1g Total Sugars 4.5g

CHAPTER 11:

SPECIAL CHAFFLE RECIPES

39. Triple Chocolate Chaffle

Preparation time: 5 minutes

Difficulty level: Medium

Cooking Time:7–9 Minutes

Servings: 2

Ingredients:

- Batter
- 4 eggs

- 4 ounces cream cheese, softened
- 1 ounce dark unsweetened chocolate, melted
- 1 teaspoon vanilla extract
- 5 tablespoons almond flour
- 3 tablespoons cocoa powder
- 1½ teaspoons baking powder
- ¼ cup dark unsweetened chocolate chips
- Other
- 2 tablespoons butter to brush the waffle maker

Directions:

1. Preheat the waffle maker.
2. Add the eggs and cream cheese to a bowl and stir with a wire whisk until just combined.
3. Add the vanilla extract and mix until combined.
4. Stir in the almond flour, cocoa powder, and baking powder and mix until combined.

5. Add the chocolate chips and stir.
6. Brush the heated waffle maker with butter and add a few tablespoons of the batter. Close the lid and cook for about 8 minutes depending on your waffle maker. Serve and enjoy.

Nutrition: Calories 385, fat 33 g, carbs 10.6 g, sugar 0.7 g, Protein 12.g, sodium 199 mg

40. Keto Coffee Chaffles

Preparation time: 10 minutes

Difficulty level: Medium

Cooking Time:5 minutes

Servings: 2

Ingredients:

- 1 tbsp. almond flour
- 1 tbsp. instant coffee
- 1/2 cup cheddar cheese
- ½ tsp baking powder
- 1 large egg

Directions:

1. Preheat waffle iron and grease with cooking spray
2. Meanwhile, in a small mixing bowl, mix together all ingredients and ½ cup cheese.
3. Pour 1/8 cup cheese in a waffle maker and then pour the mixture in the center of greased waffle.

4. Again, sprinkle cheese on the batter.
5. Close the waffle maker.
6. Cook chaffles for about 4-5 minutes Utes until cooked and crispy.
7. Once chaffles are cooked, remove and enjoy!

Nutrition: Protein: 26% 47 kcal Fat: 69% 125 kcal Carbohydrates: 5% 9 kcal

41. Breakfast Spinach Ricotta Chaffles

Preparation time: 8 minutes

Difficulty level: Medium

Cooking Time: 28 Minutes **Servings:** 2

Ingredients:

- 4 oz frozen spinach, thawed, squeezed dry
- 1 cup ricotta cheese
- 2 eggs, beaten
- ½ tsp garlic powder
- ¼ cup finely grated Pecorino Romano cheese
- ½ cup finely grated mozzarella cheese
- Salt and freshly ground black pepper to taste

Directions:

1. Preheat the waffle iron.
2. In a medium bowl, mix all the ingredients.

3. Open the iron, lightly grease with cooking spray and spoon in a quarter of the mixture.
4. Close the iron and cook until brown and crispy, 7 minutes.
5. Remove the chaffle onto a plate and set aside. Make three more chaffles with the remaining mixture. Allow cooling and serve afterward.

Nutrition: Calories 1Fats 13.15gCarbs 5.06gNet Carbs 4.06gProtein 12.79g

42. Yogurt Chaffle

Preparation time: 8 minutes

Cooking Time: 10 Minutes

Difficulty level: Easy

Servings: 2

Ingredients:

- 1/2 cup mozzarella cheese, shredded
- 1/2 cup cheddar cheese, shredded
- 1 egg
- 2 tbsps. ground almonds
- 1 tsp. psyllium husk
- ¼ tsp. baking powder
- 1 tbsp. Greek yogurt
- TOPPING
- 1 scoop heavy cream, frozen
- 1 scoop raspberry puree, frozen

- 2 raspberries

Directions:

1. Mix together all of the chaffle ingredients and heat up your Waffle Maker.
2. Let the batter stand for 5 minutes Utes.
3. Spray waffles maker with cooking spray.
4. spread some cheese on chaffle maker and pour chaffle mixture in heart shape Belgian waffle maker.
5. Close the lid and cook for about 4-minutesutes. For serving, scoop frozen cream and puree in the middle of chaffle.
6. Top with a raspberry. Serve and enjoy!

Nutrition: Protein: 31% 41 kcal Fat: 66% 88 kcal Carbohydrates: 3% 4 kcal

43. Chaffles With Caramelized Apples And Yogurt

Preparation time: 10 minutes **Cooking Time:** 10 Minutes

Difficulty level: Easy **Servings:** 2

Ingredients:

- 1 tablespoon unsalted butter
- 1 tablespoon golden brown sugar
- 1 Granny Smith apple, cored and thinly sliced
- 1 pinch salt
- 2 whole-grain frozen waffles, toasted
- 1/2 cup mozzarella cheese, shredded
- 1/4 cup Yoplait® Original French Vanilla yogurt

Direction

- Melt the butter in a large skillet over medium-high heat until starting to brown. Add mozzarella cheese and stir well.

- Add the sugar, apple slices and salt and cook, stirring frequently, until apples are softened and tender, about 6 to 9 minutes.
- Put one warm waffle each on a plate, top each with yogurt and apples. Serve warm.

Nutrition: Calories: 240 calories Total Fat: 10.4 g Cholesterol: 54 mg Sodium: 226 mg Total Carbohydrate: 33.8 g Protein: 4.7 g

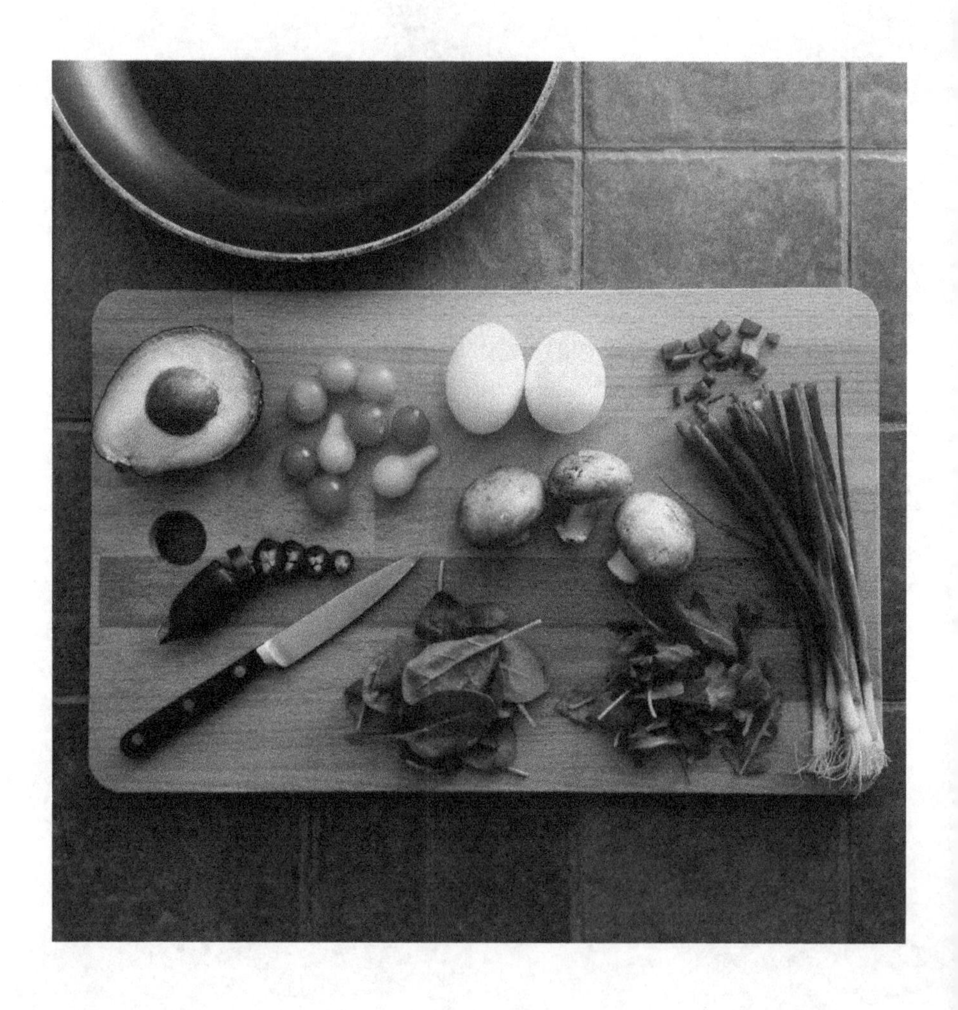

CHAPTER 12:

OTHER KETO CHAFFLES

44. Shrimp Avocado Chaffle Sandwich

Preparation time: 8 minutes

Difficulty level: Easy

Cooking Time: 32 Minutes

Servings: 2

Ingredients:

- 2 cups shredded mozzarella cheese
- 4 large eggs
- ½ tsp curry powder
- ½ tsp oregano

- Shrimp Sandwich Filling:
- 1-pound raw shrimp (peeled and deveined)
- 1 large avocado (diced)
- 4 slices cooked bacon
- 2 tbsp sour cream
- ½ tsp paprika
- 1 tsp Cajun seasoning
- 1 tbsp olive oil
- ¼ cup onion (finely chopped)
- 1 red bell pepper (diced)

Directions:

1. Plug the waffle maker to preheat it and spray it with a non-stick cooking spray.
2. Break the eggs into a mixing bowl and beat. Add the cheese, oregano and curry. Mix until the ingredients are well combined.

3. Pour an appropriate amount of the batter into the waffle maker and spread out the batter to the edges to cover all the holes on the waffle maker. This should make 8 mini waffles.
4. Close the waffle maker and cook for about minutes or according to your waffle maker's settings.
5. After the cooking cycle, use a silicone or plastic utensil to remove the chaffle from the waffle maker.
6. Repeat step 3 to 5 until you have cooked all the batter into chaffles.
7. Heat up the olive oil in a large skillet over medium to high heat.
8. Add the shrimp and cook until the shrimp is pink and tender.
9. Remove the skillet from heat and use a slotted spoon to transfer the shrimp to a paper towel lined plate to drain for a few minutes.

10. Put the shrimp in a mixing bowl. Add paprika and Cajun seasoning. Toss until the shrimps are all coated with seasoning.
11. To assemble the sandwich, place one chaffle on a flat surface and spread some sour cream over it. Layer some shrimp, onion, avocado, diced pepper and one slice of bacon over it. Cover with another chaffle.
12. Repeat step 10 until you have assembled all the ingredients into sandwiches.
13. Serve and enjoy.

Nutrition: Fat 32.1g 41% Carbohydrate 10.8g 4% Sugars 2.5g Protein 44.8g

45. Cuban Pork Sandwich

Preparation time: 5 minutes

Difficulty level: Easy

Cooking Time: 10 Minutes

Servings: 2

Ingredients:

- Sandwich Filling:
- 25 g swiss cheese (sliced)
- 2 ounces cooked deli ham (thinly sliced)
- 3 slices pickle chips
- ½ tbsp Dijon mustard
- ½ tbsp mayonnaise
- 3 ounces pork roast
- 1 tsp paprika
- 1 stalk celery (diced)
- Chaffle:

- 1 tsp baking powder
- 1 large egg (beaten)
- 1 tbsp full-fat Greek yogurt
- 4 tbsp mozzarella cheese
- 1 tbsp almond flour

Directions:

1. Preheat the oven to 350°F and grease a baking sheet.
2. Plug the waffle maker to preheat it and spray it with a non-stick cooking spray.
3. In a mixing bowl, combine the almond flour, cheese and baking powder.
4. Add the egg and yogurt. Mix until the ingredients are well combined.
5. Fill the waffle maker with an appropriate amount of the batter and spread the batter to the edges to cover all the holes on the waffle maker.

6. Close the waffle maker and cook the waffle until it is crispy. That will take about 5 minutes. The time may vary in some waffle makers.
7. After the cooking cycle, remove the chaffle from the waffle maker with a plastic or silicone utensil.
8. Repeat step 4 to 6 until you have cooked all the batter into chaffles.
9. In a small mixing bowl, combine the mustard, oregano and mayonnaise.
10. Brush the mustard-mayonnaise mixture over the surface of both chaffles.
11. Layer the pork, ham, pickles and celery over one of the chaffles. Layer the cheese slices on top and cover it with the second chaffle.
12. Place it on the baking sheet. Place it in oven and bake until the cheese melts. You can place a heavy stainless

place over the chaffle to make the sandwich come out flat after baking

13. After the baking cycle, remove the chaffle sandwich from the oven and let it cool for a few minutes.
14. Serve warm and enjoy.

Nutrition: Fat 52.3g 67% Carbohydrate 17.3g 6% Sugars 2.7g Protein 82.6g

46. Garlic Mayo Vegan Chaffles

Preparation time: 8 minutes

Servings: 2

Difficulty level: Easy

Cooking Time: 5minutes

Ingredients:

- 1 tbsp. chia seeds
- 2 ½ tbsps. water
- ¼ cup low carb vegan cheese
- 2 tbsps. coconut flour
- 1 cup low carb vegan cream cheese, softened
- 1 tsp. garlic powder
- pinch of salt
- 2 tbsps. vegan garlic mayo for topping

Directions:

1. Preheat your square waffle maker.

2. In a small bowl, mix chia seeds and water, let it stand for 5 minutes Utes.
3. Add all ingredients to the chia seeds mixture and mix well.
4. Pour vegan chaffle batter in a greased waffle maker
5. Close the waffle maker and cook for about 3-minutesutes.
6. Once chaffles are cooked, remove from the maker.
7. Top with garlic mayo and pepper.
8. Enjoy!

Nutrition: Protein: 32% 42 kcal Fat: 63% 82 kcal Carbohydrates: 5% 6 kcal

47. Almond Butter Chaffle

Preparation time: 8 minutes

Difficulty level: Easy

Cooking Time: 20 Minutes

Servings: 2

Ingredients:

- 2 eggs (beaten)
- 3 tsp granulated swerve sweetener
- 4 tbsp almond flour
- ½ tsp vanilla extract
- ½ cup grated mozzarella cheese
- ½ cup parmesan cheese
- 1/8 tsp allspice
- Almond Butter Filling:
- ½ tsp vanilla extract
- 4 tbsp almond butter

- 2 tbsp butter (melted)
- 2 tbsp swerve sweetener
- 1/8 tsp nutmeg

Directions:

1. Plug the waffle maker to preheat it and spray it with a non-stick cooking spray.
2. In a mixing bowl, combine the mozzarella, allspice, almond flour, and swerve sweetener. Add the egg and vanilla extract and mix until the ingredients are well combined.
3. Sprinkle some parmesan cheese over the waffle maker.
4. Pour an appropriate amount of the batter into the waffle and spread out the batter to cover all the holes on the waffle maker.
5. Sprinkle some parmesan over the batter.

6. Close the waffle maker and cook for about 5 minutes or according to your waffle maker's settings.
7. After the cooking cycle, use a plastic or silicone utensil to remove the chaffle from the waffle maker. Transfer the chaffle to a wire rack to cool.
8. Repeat step 3 to 7 until you have cooked all the batter into chaffles.
9. For the filling, combine butter, almond butter, swerve, vanilla and nutmeg. Mix until the mixture is smooth and fluffy.
10. Spread the cream over the surface of one chaffle and cover the with another chaffle. Repeat until you have filled all the chaffles.
11. Serve and enjoy.

Nutrition: Fat 54.8g 70% Carbohydrate 18.4g7% Sugars 3.2g Protein 29.7g

48. Cauliflower Rice Chaffle

Preparation time: 9 minutes

Servings: 2

Difficulty level: Easy

Cooking Time: 8 Minutes

Ingredients:

- 1 cup cauliflower rice
- ¼ tsp salt or to taste
- 1 tbsp melted butter
- 1 egg
- ¼ tsp nutmeg
- ¼ tsp cinnamon
- ¼ tsp garlic powder
- 1/8 tsp ground black pepper or to taste
- 1/8 tsp white pepper or to taste
- ¼ tsp Italian seasoning

- ½ cup shredded parmesan cheese
- ½ cup shredded mozzarella cheese
- Garnish:
- Chopped green onions

Directions:

1. Pour ¼ of the parmesan cheese into a blender, add the mozzarella cheese, egg, salt, nutmeg, butter, cinnamon, garlic powder, black pepper, white pepper, Italian seasoning and cauliflower.
2. Add the egg and blend until you form a smooth batter.
3. Plug the waffle maker and preheat it. Spray the waffle maker with a non-stick spray.
4. Sprinkle about tbsp of the remaining parmesan cheese on top of the waffle maker.
5. Fill the waffle maker with ¼ of the batter and spread out the batter to cover all the holes on the waffle

maker. Sprinkle some shredded parmesan over the batter.

6. Close the lid of the waffle maker and cook for about 4 to 5 minutes or according to your waffle maker's settings.
7. After the cooking cycle, remove the waffle with a rubber or silicone utensil.
8. Repeat step 4 to 7 until you have cooked all the batter into chaffles.
9. Serve and enjoy.

Nutrition: Fat 15.8g 20% .Carbohydrate 6.2g 2% .Sugars 2.4g. Protein 15g

CHAPTER 13:

CHAFFLE MEAT RECIPES

49. Chicken Taco Chaffle

Preparation time: 10 minutes

Difficulty level: Easy **Cooking Time:** 15 Minutes

Servings: 2

Ingredients:

- Batter
- 4 eggs
- 2 cups grated provolone cheese
- 6 tablespoons almond flour
- 2½ teaspoons baking powder

- Salt and pepper to taste
- Chicken topping
- 2 tablespoons olive oil
- ½ pound ground chicken
- Salt and pepper to taste
- 1 garlic clove, minced
- 2 teaspoons dried oregano
- Other
- 2 tablespoons butter to brush the waffle maker
- 2 tablespoons freshly chopped spring onion for garnishing

Directions:

1. Preheat the waffle maker.
2. Add the eggs, grated provolone cheese, almond flour, baking powder and salt and pepper to a bowl. Mix until just combined. Brush the heated waffle maker

with cooking spray and add a few tablespoons of the batter.

3. Close the lid and cook for about 7–9 minutes depending on your waffle maker. Meanwhile, heat the olive oil in a nonstick pan over medium heat and start cooking the ground chicken.
4. Season with salt and pepper and stir in the minced garlic and dried oregano. Cook for 10 minutes.
5. Add some of the cooked ground chicken to each chaffle and serve with freshly chopped spring onion.

Nutrition: Calories 584, fat 44 g, carbs 6.4 g, sugar 0.8 g, Protein 41.3g, sodium 737 mg

50. Italian Chicken And Basil Chaffle

Preparation time: 10 minutes **Difficulty level:** Easy

Cooking Time: 7–9 Minutes **Servings:** 2

Ingredients:

- Batter
- ½ pound ground chicken
- 4 eggs 3 tablespoons tomato sauce
- Salt and pepper to taste
- 1 cup grated mozzarella cheese
- 1 teaspoon dried oregano
- 3 tablespoons freshly chopped basil leaves
- ½ teaspoon dried garlic
- Other
- 2 tablespoons butter to brush the waffle maker
- ¼ cup tomato sauce for serving
- 1 tablespoon freshly chopped basil for serving

Directions:

1. Preheat the waffle maker.
2. Add the ground chicken, eggs and tomato sauce to a bowl and season with salt and pepper.
3. Add the mozzarella cheese and season with dried oregano, freshly chopped basil and dried garlic.
4. Mix until fully combined and batter forms.
5. Brush the heated waffle maker with butter and add a few tablespoons of the chaffle batter.
6. Close the lid and cook for about 7–9 minutes depending on your waffle maker.
7. Repeat with the rest of the batter.
8. Serve with tomato sauce and freshly chopped basil on top.

Nutrition: Calories 250, fat 15.7 g, carbs 2.5 g, sugar 1.5 g, Protein 24.5 g, sodium 334 mg

CONCLUSION

In the low-carb world, the word 'CHAFFLE' appeared and took the social media by storm. The waffle maker became the need of every keto kitchen and individuals following ketogenic diet found their new love. This new addition in the keto diet is not only healthy but the possibilities to experiment with new recipes are countless.
Furthermore, it has also made it easy for keto followers to follow their diet and controlling their cravings for flour based foods. In simple words, chaffles are the low-carb waffles – they are called chaffle because cheese is used as their base ingredient. Cheese and waffle by combining these words you will get the delicious chaffles.
Another benefit that we offer? We explain routines that you can do for yourself to make this diet last longer for you and to benefit your body better as a result. Routines are very important and can be a big help to your body but also your spirit and your mind.
This will help you utilize the diet better, and you will be able to improve with it as well as have it become easier for you to handle. You want to stay healthy and make sure that your body is able to do what it needs to.
As with anything, we have put a strong emphasis on the fact that if anything feels wrong or unnatural, you will need to see a doctor to make sure that you are safe and that your body can handle this diet. Use the knowledge in this book to have amazing recipes and learn how to prepare amazing meals for you.

How to Clean and Maintain the Waffle Maker

Make sure that it is not hot before you clean the waffle or chaffle maker. But clean it as soon as it is cool enough.

1. Use a damp cloth or paper towel for wiping away the crumbs.
2. Soak up the excess oil drips on your grid plates.
3. Wipe the exterior with the damp cloth or paper towel.
4. Pour a few drops of cooking oil on the batter to remove the stubborn batter drips. Wipe it away after this.
5. You can wash the cooking plates in soapy warm water. Rinse them clean.

6. Ensure that the waffle maker is completely dry before storing it.

Waffle Maker Maintenance Tips

Remember these simple tips and your waffle maker will serve you for a long time.

- Instruction manual should be well read before you use it for the first time.
- Only a light cooking oil coating is required for nonstick waffle makers.
- Grease the grid with only a little amount of oil if you see the waffles sticking.
- Never use metal or sharp tools to scrape off the batter or to remove the cooked waffles. You may end up scratching the surface and damaging it.
- Do not submerge your electric waffle maker in water.

Chaffles can be frozen and processed, so a large proportion can be made and stored for quick and extremely fast meals. If you don't have a waffle maker, just cook the mixture like a pancake in a frying pan, or even cooler, in a fryer-pan. They won't get all the fluffy sides to achieve like you're using a waffle maker, but they're definitely going to taste great.

Depending on which cheese you choose, the carbs and net calorie number can shift a little bit. However, in general, whether you use real, whole milk cheese, chaffles are completely carb-free.

For up to a month, chaffles will be frozen. However, defrosting them absorbs plenty of moist, which makes it difficult to get their crisp again. Chaffles are rich in fat and moderate in protein and low in carb. Chaffle is a very well established and popular technique to hold people on board.

And the chaffles are more durable and better than most forms of keto bread. "What a high-carb diet you may be desirous of. A nonstick waffle maker is something that makes life easier, and it's a trade-off that's happy to embrace for our wellbeing.

CPSIA information can be obtained
at www.ICGtesting.com
Printed in the USA
BVHW090805120521
607041BV00005B/1068

9 781802 672015